BEING SMOKE FREE IS YOUR CHOICE

MICHAEL YEAGER, B.A., LCDC, CHT., CAS, CTC

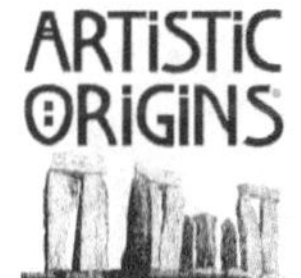

Books by Michael Yeager,
B.A., LCDC, CHt., CAS, CTC

12+2 Steps Young People in Recovery

Coming Soon

Thoughts of Solitude an Interpretation

Resolving Death and Non-Death Related Losses

Evidence-Based Rapid Resolution Therapy, i.e.,
It does not have to take a lifetime to heal

An Approach to Addiction Treatment

A Near-Death Experience and After

Being Smoke Free is Your Choice by Michael Yeager, B.A., LCDC, CHt., CAS, CTC

Published by Artistic Origins

Cover design: deborahola: https://www.fiverr.com/deborahola

Interior layout by Dawn G. Ireland

ISBN 9781940385389 (eBook)

ISBN 9781940385396 (paperback)

Michael Yeager, B.A., LCDC, CHt., CAS, CTC

9525 Katy Freeway, Suite 428, Houston, Texas 77024

Please visit my websites: For Counseling: www.holisticouncil.org and

For Mental Health Professionals CEU's Home-study Courses
www.ceuprocourses.com

Sign up for my newsletter at: ceuinfo@ceuinfo.com

Wholesale discounts: contact the author.

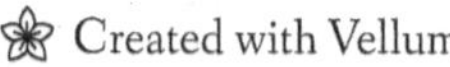

Books by Michael Yeager,
B.A., LCDC, CHt., CAS, CTC

12+2 Steps Young People in Recovery

Coming Soon

Thoughts of Solitude an Interpretation

Resolving Death and *Non-Death Related Losses*

Evidence-Based Rapid Resolution Therapy, i.e.,
It does not have to take a lifetime to heal

An Approach to Addiction Treatment

A *Near-Death Experience* and After

Being Smoke Free is Your Choice by Michael Yeager, B.A., LCDC, CHt., CAS, CTC

Published by Artistic Origins

Cover design: deborahola: https://www.fiverr.com/deborahola

Interior layout by Dawn G. Ireland

ISBN 9781940385389 (eBook)

ISBN 9781940385396 (paperback)

Michael Yeager, B.A., LCDC, CHt., CAS, CTC

9525 Katy Freeway, Suite 428, Houston, Texas 77024

Please visit my websites: For Counseling: www.holisticcouncil.org and

For Mental Health Professionals CEU's Home-study Courses
www.ceuprocourses.com

Sign up for my newsletter at: ceuinfo@ceuinfo.com

Wholesale discounts: contact the author.

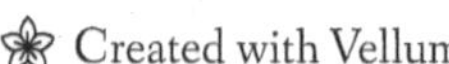

ACKNOWLEDGMENTS

A great cover says it all. Many thanks to Deborahola on the Fiverr website (https://www.fiverr.com/deborahola). She created an outstanding cover!

My thanks goes out to Dawn Greenfield Ireland, a very professional editor. She offered helpful suggestions, and the comments she made helped me to add more depth and clarity to the book. I felt comfortable with her input and insight into the topic. I look forward to ongoing support and help with my other books.

I also want to thank Kathy Herranen for her initial editing work on this book. I appreciate her input and comments she made to help me get started.

I thank everyone who I have ever known whether I judged the relationship good or bad.

All my teachers—my parents: Frances and Eileen Yeager,

my siblings, cousins, aunts, uncles, drug using acquaintances, sober friends, and acquaintances.

ACTIONS APPRECIATED

Please leave a review on Goodreads, Amazon and my website! Reviews help authors get recognized, get the word out and sell more books.

ENDORSEMENT

Wow, amazing! January 26, 2007, Roger and I were smoking cigarettes and about to go into Michael Yeager's home/office to be hypnotized. We came out 60 minutes later and neither one of us has smoked since. The power of the subconscious mind accessed through specific small steps is truly amazing.

Thank you, Michael, for helping us create new beliefs and behaviors that have changed our lives. I have to say that when you told us to write down our beliefs about how our lives would be worse off as a non-smoker, just might be better as a non-smoker and the triggers that associated us to smoking and bring them with us really did make a difference. Your wisdom is incredible.

Kathleen & Roger B

TRUTH VS FALSEHOOD

The Truth (what happened)

"Just the facts man just the facts"

The Story (what I tell myself-
assumptions, guess work-
personalization's-victimizations-lies,
made up fantasies that I settle on
and call that is what happened.

No truth – No Facts – Just my Story.

Then I live as if my story is true, and it
colors the facts so all I can see is my
made-up story –

that I call the truth which is

just my story.

CHAPTER 1

Being Smoke Free is the easiest thing I have ever done

This statement will be turned into your reality when you apply the principles discussed in this book. I will discuss change in behavior in possibly a way that you have not considered before. I encourage each of you to pay close attention and contemplate every idea. Your success depends upon your accepting and acting on these exercises.

Be willing to break out of an old belief pattern, i.e., that of seeing, speaking, thinking, and acting like a smoker. This journey out of an old belief can, and probably will, be met with resistance, fear, rejection, denial, and skepticism. Note from the onset that these reactions are to be expected whenever change occurs. You are challenging old, stable, nurtured beliefs about yourself, and these beliefs have most likely been with you for a long time.

It is as if the ideas are always running in your head regardless of your conscious awareness of them or not. To borrow a phrase from *The Forum*: "Already-Always Listening." For those of you feeling forced by another or by your failing health and are angry about this, the same is true. No one or nothing can force you to do anything. That is why the idea of *choice* is so important. You may find that if you choose to be a non-smoker you are choosing the best of two evils regardless, it is our choice.

As you continue with the exercises, pay close attention to how you respond to the ideas. Notice how you feel when you go through the motions. This self-awareness is especially important because as you acknowledge more about yourself, the more powerful and in control you will become.

This idea came about as I looked at the messages I gave to myself about smoking and everything else in my life. One thing I noticed was that I never lied to myself about anything. If I told myself that something was going to be a certain way at my deepest belief level, then that is the way it turned out. This made me look beyond the surface messages and go deeper within my mind, and I could only accomplish this by taking the time to notice the self-talk that is with me day in and day out. I had to force myself to pay attention to that chatter.

This discipline required a work effort of three to five-seconds, 10 to 20 times a day. As I heard the dialogue in my head, I noticed I was persistent in my behavior to match the self-talk deep within me. That caused a sigh of relief because now I could honestly say that I had gotten out of life exactly what I wanted. As Maxwell Maltz stated in his book *Psycho-Cybernetics,* "Humans are incapable of failing. All we can do is succeed at producing results that are consistent with our deepest level of beliefs."

My life totally paralleled my deepest thoughts. I also noticed that this difference in the level of thoughts caused my frustration and confusion. The surface message I saw was, *I want to stop smoking*, while the underlying message I sent myself was, *I cannot stop smoking because ...*

The list of "because's" was extremely long and had a lot of thought energy attached to them. What this revelation showed me was that I had inconsistent thoughts that I could not stop, and I wanted to stop, but I could not because, by very consistent behavior (I remained a smoker). Therefore, I was responsible for my ongoing smoking because my thoughts and behaviors matched the deepest levels of my mind.

Can you imagine how free I felt at this point? If I really was constant in both thought and action at one level of thought, then all I had to do to change my behavior was to replace the old message with a new message. I had to bring the surface message, *What I think I want* down to the deeper message of *What I manifest in my life.*

First, I had to become aware of the old messages/beliefs.

Then I had to get to know the ways they presented themselves to me in my life.

(Specificity) I needed to really hear what they were before I could change them.

This process of identity was one I did not like because I had to become very honest with myself, and honesty can be very painful. It did not make me happy knowing that I had put a lot of energy into my excuses for why I could not quit smoking. It was embarrassing to admit that I did not know how to function in life without a cigarette. If this was the price I had to pay to stop smoking, then I was willing to pay the price.

Through the self-awareness exercises, discussed in these pages, I would not be willing to stop smoking for a negative reason like failing health, coughing, smelling like smoke and nicotine, having a foul taste in my mouth, or heat in my lungs. Even though I knew these things, and realized they affected my life, and I did not like the effects, I still had not and could not quit.

Knowing this about myself, I decided I would look for a positive reason to stop, like, *I Love Me.* I was aware from psychology, counseling, success-motivation courses, and my short salesmen career that goal setting was especially important. If I had a goal to shoot for, then I could stay motivated to achieve it.

My goal was set far enough in advance that I thought I could achieve my desired result. I will say now, and more later about that, I missed my first goal. On my 30th day (the initial goal date) of my smoking cessation program, I was walking in downtown Denver and a lady I knew from a salesman's organization I belonged to, Salesman with a Purpose (SWAP), saw me and asked me if the day before was supposed to be my last cigarette.

And was not today then my 1st smoke free date? I said *Yes*, and I was still smoking. 1,000+ excuses followed for still smoking on my initial stop date. We talked some more and then she asked me if I believed all that stuff I talked about, i.e., goal setting, personal power, goal achievement, etc.

My pride swelled up, and I said *yes.* She then said something that emphatically changed my life. She said, well then do it! She turned and just walked off.

It occurred to me that my mind just needed more time to accept the new vision and kept up with my affirmations, imagery, self-talk, etc. All judgement-free. Because of the positive work I had done on myself to get to the first date, I simply set another goal and was successful on the second attempt 26 days later. Because of this I found that my mind would accept any new message I gave it. All I needed to do was repeat it often enough for my mind to catch on and accept it.

Persistence

In my quiet time, I noticed I had a mental image of myself as a smoker. I could not seem to see myself as a non-smoker. It had been too long to remember what I was like, how I felt, smelled, and acted as a non-smoker.

As I was discussing this with a friend, I said, "*I just can't imagine what I'll feel like as a non-smoker.*"

He said, "*You'll probably feel good!*"

Now I had something to relate to; now I knew what it was like to feel good. So, when I created an image of myself as a *non-smoker*, I created a mental image of myself feeling good, smelling fresh, and acting comfortable, basically using general terms I could relate to. This allowed me to see myself as I wanted to be seen, or live in the solution.

Another important decision for myself was, if I was going to become a non-smoker, I had to become someone who refused to give smokers a bad time. Not smoking was my choice, so that is all it was—a choice. It was my choice to not be offended by smokers, and under no circumstances would I become an obnoxious non-smoker.

Only you are responsible for every aspect of your life. All decisions and choices are yours to make. The sooner you accept this, the faster you will affect a lasting change in any area of your life.

When you own your responsibility and your thoughts, then you can choose to do whatever you want to do with your behavior. This acceptance begins in the mind.

We hold all our perceptions, ideas, concepts, facts, aspects of who we are, what we think we can and cannot do, how we see ourselves in this life, our self-concept, and how we perceive the world around us inside our mind. Our mind is our window to our reality. All our decisions are based on our unique belief systems, which are made up of how we choose to perceive reality.

If you agree and accept the concept that you are responsible for how you experience everything that happens to you, then you see and understand that you choose how you perceive reality. Therefore, it holds true that you can change your perception about you as a smoker to that of a non-smoker.

Once you change your perception, then you will be able to change your actions. We exhibit the behavior that is thought about the most at the deepest levels of our minds. If we think that not smoking will be a very tough thing to do, then it will. Likewise, if we think it will be easy, then it will. We are in control of our thoughts and actions. A statement of our strength is our willingness to confront and change our belief and behavior.

CHAPTER 2

It is necessary to complete the exercises and follow the instructions in the book. I know that you have:

1. Tried to stop smoking in the past, or
2. Never tried to stop smoking before.

You most likely have a preconceived notion about the success or failure of this course. I assume you expect success and that you will work the steps of the course as if it will work for you. This expectation is particularly important because it helps lay the groundwork for how successful you will be. It is necessary that you understand the ideas laid out in the course are not theory. They are reports of action taken. As Maxwell Maltz stated in his book *Psycho-Cybernetics,* "You will be a success no matter what you do." We always get what we think about the most. We automatically manifest the behavior that is most closely aligned with our inner-most thoughts.

The exercises are tools you can use to change your thoughts about you as a smoker to that of a non-smoker. They are simple, require some time, but typically require you to make a conscious commitment to do them. Repetition is the key to learning. Yes, this is an old saying, and it is true.

At present, you, as a smoker, are, or have given yourself messages to reinforce your smoking, remember repetition is the key to learning i.e.,

- To stop smoking will be impossible.
- I'll get fat.
- I'll become unbearable to be with without a cigarette.
- I don't have the willpower.
- I need something in my mouth to calm me down.
- I can't manage my stress without a cigarette.
- I don't know what I'll do with my hands.

All these messages are of your own creation. They are your self-imposed blocks and barriers to effecting change. These messages, and many, many more that you continuously repeat, enable you to demonstrate the behavior of a smoker who believes it will be difficult at best to stop.

It is important for you to be aware of all your self-talk about why you can't quit. Notice the energy you put into your statements. Observe the level of expectancy for success you put into your statements. Look at your backlog of data to prove your point. Notice the length of time you have given yourself the same messages. It is important that you reflect on this information so that you can realize who you are in relationship to it.

You are basically identifying the problem for you right now. We must start with a foundation, and this gives you that basis to work from. See the importance repetition has played in helping you achieve success in the maintenance of your smoking behavior. All these things, actions, and thoughts you hold on to allow you to defend your behavior as a smoker and justify to yourself why you can't quit. This energy can be turned around and used to support a new behavior—being smoke free.

CHOICE IS THE KEY HERE—YOU can choose to be smoke free. The statement of choice frees you from the habit. By believing you can choose to be smoke free, or to smoke makes you responsible for your behavior. The acceptance of the idea of choice puts you in a position to effect change. Once you own an aspect of your behavior, then you can do something about it. All the excuses must be cast aside. You can no longer play victim to circumstances and expect to easily stop.

By telling yourself, repeatedly, that you can choose to stop smoking will eventually help you to believe this. It is critical that you choose to stop smoking for a positive reason, like *I Love Myself,* or some other positive growth-oriented phrase. You have known for years all the negatives about smoking, and they have not helped you stop or stay stopped.

People can generally come up with the *So what?* Or *it can't happen to me* attitude when it comes to things like cancer, black lung, emphysema, and shortness of breath. We can easily discount these things: the smell of smoke, or coughing up last night's smoke. We have known this stuff about the effects of smoking for years, and it has not been a sufficient deterrent to stop yet, so why should it work for you now?

Therefore, I believe if you have a positive, simple phrase, then the results will be positive. The upbeat, *I love me,* infers I am showing a caring action to myself which differs from the negative of: *If I don't quit, terrible things will happen to me.* So, in effect, you are not running from something; you are choosing to accept something good. It has to do with how you think about it.

Remember, this course is designed to help you see your relationship to smoking differently. The idea of how changing your thinking can change your actions is an important concept for you to understand. I ask that you do not judge yourself as a smoker, and not judge smoking behavior. If you judge, you risk putting energy into the problem vs the solution.

By refusing to judge, you are better able to keep the idea of choice uppermost in your mind. Also, by not judging your smoking or not smoking behavior, there is no emotional charge in either direction, so you can exercise your choice much easier —the flow can be there for you. By avoiding the good/bad issue (dualistic thinking), you will also be less prone to becoming an obnoxious non-smoker. We all know what it is like to be judged by a non-smoker. It adds fuel to the fire.

IT IS PARTICULARLY important to know that you are making a choice to be smoke free, and that is that. We are simply exercising our choice—we do not have to justify our choice by forcing others to do as we do, or by making up a fantasy story about the difficulty we are surely to face when we stop. We do not need to place our energy on smoking or not because we can end up with us being resentful, which can lead back to smoking or other unloving behavior. When you passively accept your choice to be smoke free, you no longer must put any emotional energy into the smoking issue.

By staying away from this energy and the smoking issue you take the action of being smoke free now; there will be no more emotional charge to it. There will be no desire to smoke or not to smoke. It will simply incorporate what you do into your entire belief system.

There is no need for all the *crutches* for not smoking, like toothpicks, bubblegum, the something in your mouth to satisfy this craving. The craving to have something in your mouth is the same craving as smoking. It keeps the idea of *you must have something in your mouth to be satisfied* alive. If that craving exists within you, you are trapped into the idea of having a cigarette. Shrink this idea that you need anything at all in your mouth until it no longer exists.

The mind works very mechanically. If you continue to put a toothpick in your mouth, or if you chew gum after meals, or similar things like hard candy, you are still thinking you need a cigarette. This will keep the whole idea of the habit alive. So, by placing no energy at all into the non-smoking issue, you will not need these other *tools* to kill the smoking habit. As you can see, the habit involves much more than the cigarette.

Now you need to decide when to stop smoking. Set a date 30 to 60 days from today. You have smoked for some time now, so 30 to 60 days will be enough time to desensitize your image of yourself as a smoker to that of a non-smoker.

The exercises in this course will enable you to stop on the date with no problems, no discomfort or annoyance, no weight gain, or negative personality change. If you follow the instructions and if you do the exercises daily, you will easily accomplish your choice to be smoke free.

YOUR BRAIN NEEDS time for the new messages to replace the old messages. Do not rush through this process. It took years of unconscious information to get you to believe, as you do now. It will take a short time to consciously change the self-talk. Take it easy, but do it! Having a concrete date to shoot for will keep you headed in a definite direction. The date needs to be far enough in advance for you to believe you can achieve success by that time, but no longer than 30 or 60 days. It gives you a framework to work within as far as time expectancy and energy. Having a goal to shoot for enables your mind to go in a specific direction to look for a specific goal to make everything very concrete and easy to obtain.

When I set my first date, there was a 30-day period. I missed the first date, and I simply rescheduled and was able to effect stopping smoking on the second date I set. So, it took me a total of 58 days to effectively show the desired result. Not smoking, where I was comfortable, with no weight gain, where I had a very pleasing personality. In fact, it was a simple thing for me to do, just like I had told myself during that entire period.

What you need to understand is that all of us are different. We all have a distinctive level of resistance to change. There doesn't seem to be a way to measure this difference, but I know that hypnotic courses and motivational books all refer to 30 to 60 days of daily repetition, affirming the new message regularly before the behavior is demonstrated.

The mind simply needs time—its own time—to absorb the new message and then produce the desired result. So, once you have the date, it is important that you continue the messages daily and become very persistent. Do not overwork yourself during this process, but keep a regimen or a schedule of daily repetition many times throughout the day. Use your thoughts and behavioral smoking actions to trigger the new messages to repeat themselves.

Now that you have set your date and you understand the importance of choosing to change your behavior for some positive reason, write it out. Here is a suggestion:

I choose to stop smoking on (Date) because I love myself.

IT IS A SIMPLE, short statement that is easy for the mind to grasp. It is there and does not take any time, or relatively no time at all, to read the statement. Now you will take this card and statement and put it up so you will see and read it at least two to three dozen times a day.

Read and say them first thing in the morning, all throughout the day and again, the last thing at night.

Your subconscious does not know the difference between fact and fiction, so by giving it a message you reenforce your goal:

- You will see it as it is written down
- You will read aloud
- You will hear the message
- The message then takes root

You can also place the message on the dash of your car, on the bathroom mirror, the refrigerator, your desk—anywhere where you will glance at it and see it throughout the day, as often as you can. At these other times, it is most important that you remind your subconscious of the goal and the choice. This way, whether you are consciously or unconsciously working on the goal, action is being taken.

Action is most important—you must commit yourself to do these things:

- Write it out
  - I choose to stop smoking or be smoke free on (date) because I love myself (or some other positive motivation)
- Read it aloud
  - First thing in the morning, last thing at night
- Remind yourself throughout the day every time you engage with a smoking activity, (reaching for a cigarette, smoking, taking a drag, flicking the ashes, putting a cigarette out) by glancing at the card of your commitment.
- Do not judge your smoking or non-smoking behavior, or that of others.

If you refuse to commit to these things, then the course and the ideas presented here simply will not work. Action keeps you a smoker. Action on new thought enables you to become smoke free.

The ideas are based on:

- Decision
- Belief
- Choice
- Love of Self

- Goal Setting
- Visualization
- Repetition
- Audio and Visual Actions
- Action

It is mostly a letting go, or a passive process. As you repeat the new, or different, messages daily, simple changes are positive, with little effort on your part.

Follow the instructions and take what you get.

With the information presented in this chapter, I suggest that you re-read the information every day, two or three times a day, for this week. Just continue to absorb the information presented in this chapter. As you go through, you will get new information. But, as I stated earlier, it has taken awhile for you to get to this point, so a few more days of smoking will not hurt, anyway.

Go over and over the information previously stated, get familiar with it, allow yourself to digest it. Get comfortable knowing who you are, with finding out what is going on inside you as these new ideas are being instilled in your mind.

CHAPTER 3

This chapter will provide another tool to reinforce the additional information about yourself to incorporate into your belief system. Some lessons include:

- Use your imagination
- How to relax
- Question your belief system
- Make changes to your belief system
- Level of expectancy in your ability to change

Besides verbal messages, you also have a mental image of you as a smoker. This mental image will need to be replaced with an image of you as a non-smoker. In this exercise, you will visualize yourself as a smoker only once. Then you will see yourself as a non-smoker possessing all the qualities you desire about yourself as a non-smoker.

Your mental image of yourself remains consistent with your verbal messages and shows itself in outward action. What is going on in your outer behavior is consistent with what is going on with your inner image Harmony. Once again, you will be breaking out of your old verbal and mental image of yourself into demonstrating a new belief and behavior.

The work is the conscious effort you are willing to give the exercises daily. The conflict will be the fight you will have with yourself being unwilling, or at least reluctant, to believe the new image will be you. Remember, you have years of experience in seeing you as a smoker, and this new image will not be consistent with the old image. Expect the fight, but do the exercises!

Visualizing, or using your imagination, to create a sense or picture of yourself as a non-smoker is the nature of this exercise. Do not be bothered by the term *visualize*. It is unnecessary that you mentally see any image; some people do, some do not. Learn to trust your imagination and trust the first sense that comes up for you as you do the exercise. There is no right or wrong way. Just think about yourself in the exercise; you already know what it feels like to think about yourself, right? Go through a practice exercise, so you know beforehand just what it feels like to sense or visualize or think about what the exercise suggests.

CLOSE YOUR EYES AND RELAX. With your mind's eye, look at the wall in your house. For example, the wall where the TV is located. See for yourself what it looks like; get in touch with how you were feeling the last time you remember being in that room. Note the color of the wall, the pictures, the plants, anything that will help you know what it is like to be in that room. Now, open your eyes. You have just visualized or thought about something specific. It is as simple as that.

THOUGHTS CREATE your perception of things familiar and unfamiliar to you. Thought is energy and produces in action that which it is directed to produce. What this means is, you get exactly what you think about the most at the deepest levels. You may have noticed that sometimes you have been thinking about someone or something, and that person or thing appeared in your life by letter, phone, zoom. Coincidences or directed action by the intensity of your thoughts.

When you think of something or picture it—it can be completed through action. First, you must think about going to a movie before you can go to a movie. Likewise, you must visualize the drawings of your new home before you can have a new home. The ideas, or thoughts, create the mental blueprint necessary for you to act.

I must know where I want to go before I can take action to produce the results.

The Bible states, *as you sow, so shall you reap*. This means, from a practical point of view, that we always attract into our lives that which we think about the most, or believe in the most strongly, or basically expect on the deepest levels, and/or imagine the most vividly.

These exercises can be performed in two to three-seconds many times throughout the day. The more energy you put into it, the easier the physical action of quitting smoking forever becomes. There are basically four steps necessary to effectively visualize, or see:

1. Set the goal. The goal is important so that your mind has a specific date and a specific item to work towards. It provides a timeframe which enables

your automatic success drive within your psyche to become activated.

2. Create a truly clear idea, or picture, of you as a smoker. Then you will make this picture disappear, and see you as a non-smoker, relaxed, at ease. Now, think of you as a non-smoker in present terms. See yourself as a non-smoker. Be as detailed as you can. Take a picture of yourself not smoking, smiling, and in a relaxed position. Title it, *Relaxed, choosing to be smoke free*, and see this many times throughout the day.
3. See the image often. Bring this image to surface as often as you think about smoking, or as often as you smoke. Let the image come up every time you light up. Be sure you spend one to three minutes first thing in the morning and last thing at night seeing and sensing you as a non-smoker. Focus on it 20-30 times a day, clearly in a very gentle, loving way. It is important that you allow the image to passively be with you—to not feel like you are working hard to get it. Basically, the more passively you allow the image to be with you, the more effective it will become.
4. Give the image positive energy. Encourage yourself as a non-smoker. Get in touch with the good you feel as a non-smoker, smiling, breathing, walking, running. Sense how good you feel knowing that you are now a non-smoker. These mental images are affirmations that you constantly feed your psyche. This process puts your creative ability to work and allows you to accept the completion of your goal. Remember, if you affirm your smoking, then you smoke; if you affirm your non-smoking,

then you demonstrate smoke-free behavior. We are using affirmations daily, so since you have chosen to change your behavior, simply affirm the desired behavior for yourself. Use the affirmations to counter any negative doubt that occurs. The negatives are simply another form of affirmation. You are choosing to replace the negative affirmations of *How hard it will be*, with the more positive affirmations of *How nice it will be smoke free*. This is just a tool—an amazingly effective tool. To make your affirmation work, you need to pick it up and use it, though.

Practice Exercise

Let us do a practice exercise. Get into a very relaxed position.

Relaxation and taking time out for yourself is an especially important aspect of this exercise. Allow yourself to accept the images as they come up, and to relax and be at ease. Read through the instructions first, then follow them, or act on the instructions and see what you get.

Close your eyes and take two or three deep breaths. Let out the tension of the day. Start with the top of your head. Go through your skull and slowly relax your entire skull. Come down to your face, relax the forehead, your eyes, cheeks, mouth, and your neck.

Let your entire body slowly, slowly relax. Through your shoulders, arms, hands, fingers relax.

Relax your stomach, back, your calves, your thighs, your legs all the way down to your feet and toes. Just allow your entire body to become very, very relaxed. All is easy and peaceful.

Just relax. Know that you feel good all over.

Now create an image for yourself in your mind's eye. See yourself as a smoker. Get in touch with your behavior.

- How do you feel?
- How do you smell?
- When are you smoking the most?
- How do you act?

Get very in touch with the entire image of you as a smoker. Now, make this picture disappear. Simply choose for it not to be there. Now that it is gone, see yourself being smoke-free. See yourself extremely comfortable, at ease, having a very pleasing personality, seeing yourself at your desired weight, in perfect health. There is no desire for a cigarette; you do not have a craving—you are totally relaxed and at ease.

You do not have a desire for a cigarette at any time of day, or in any given situation. Visualize yourself anxious, nervous, unsure of yourself, angry, resentful, devastated, happy, sad, glad, upset, overwhelmed, at ease. You are totally at ease with yourself as a non-smoker. This is the image you will see from now on, or whenever you choose to close your eyes and see you.

If you would like to, you can record this message on your cellphone and play it back to yourself so that you have this verbal reinforcement going on as you allow yourself to see yourself as a non-smoker.

The purpose of the exercise is to practice putting your energy into the desired result, not the problem. The problem needs to be identified because you need to have a base to work from. But once the problem has been identified, focus your energy on the solution.

The entire course solves the problem. You will need to answer basic questions about yourself now. The success or failure of the course rides on your affirmative answers to these questions.

Regarding quitting smoking, do you believe you can be a non-smoker at the very deepest levels?

Look now, deep within, and see what response comes to the surface. What is the first response you get? Be aware of the self-talk—this clamor from within. It is a guiding force in your life, this voice or talk in your head. It is what we respond to as we live our lives. Pay attention to it. If it is not saying what you want it to say, allow yourself to go in and change it. That, again, is what the exercises are for. It is a tool for you to help change the self-talk that is going on within your head as a smoker. Then, you can see, you are consistent with this self-talk. Be aware of who you are and what you tell yourself about you.

Now, you need to know if you really want to change. For us to effect a change in any area of our lives, we will give something up about ourselves. Do you really want to give up your cough, smell, fancy lighters, the ashtrays, cigarette carriers, how you handle anxiety, fear, frustration, happiness—your image of you as a smoker? You will really have to give this entire image up. Give up your morning ritual, your after-dinner ritual, how you handle answering the telephone, or meeting new people where you sit in restaurants, on airplanes, why you cannot do certain exercises, etc. Your image of yourself will change. You need to know if you want to give it up.

A way you can see for yourself the strength of your desire will be in how much energy you put into the verbal new messages and your use of the visualization exercise. If you think of excuses why you cannot or will not do the exercises to counter the old messages, this is telling you that you really do not want to change. That is good to know because then you can spend your energy doing what you want to do. So, once again, the self-awareness is a way of freeing you up to do exactly as you please.

Likewise, if you do the verbal and visualization exercises consistently, conscientiously throughout the day to counter the old messages, then be assured that you will eventually follow the new messages with the new, desired action. We become what we think about the most—where you put the bulk of your energy. So, just by paying attention to yourself, you will know where you are and where you are going.

Expectancy in your belief, in your ability to change, is the needed emotion to carry you through to successful change. This emotion of expectation has the power to show whatever behavior you want to validate. Look back in your life, see where you have expected with all your heart a certain result—known that something would happen, only to have it happen. By consciously nurturing this expectancy, you can take charge of your life.

Be aware now of what that felt like, to know that something would happen. Get in touch with how you felt all over. Notice also what you did to feed the expectant feeling. By being aware of all these aspects, feelings, and emotions, you can recapture them for yourself and put them to use at will. This part of the course is particularly important.

Stop and think of how you have taken control of other behavioral changes in yourself. Reflect now, with your eyes open or closed, whichever works better for you, and see exactly, specifically what you did to effect the change. Big or little changes—it does not matter. The same identical process is at work. Be still now for a few minutes and reflect. Just relax and look.

Universal Law

The universal law is always at work in all situations. It is important that you see the common thread running through all these situations. The universal law works the same, no matter the issue. The law is, *as you think, so shall you become.* You create your own life as you choose it to be—free will.

Do not fight the exercises—simply allow yourself to do them. To counter the old messages, or whatever, or whenever you think about them, simply allow the new belief time to be accepted. Therefore, the message needs to be seen and heard every day many times throughout the day. It is important to see yourself as a non-smoker enjoying yourself, and to especially remain judge free of yourself for smoking or not smoking, or anyone else. As you repeat the new messages daily, then the behavior simply changes from within and there is no effort on your part. Remember that it is mostly a letting go or a passive process. You are choosing to be smoke free.

CHAPTER 4

For change to take place, you will need to get a complete and emotional picture of who you are now and who you want to be. By increasing your self-awareness, you will find the inner strength necessary to produce the desired behavioral change. As you see your new self, there will be gaps in behavior you may not know how to deal with yet. What is most important to know about these gaps is that they are natural and to be expected.

You will fill in these gaps as soon as you decide to use the creative process to its fullest with your visualizations. The action you will take is most important. See yourself doing whatever you want during these times. It is your life, so be a fantastic architect and develop yourself to your fullest extent.

There may be a sense of loss that accompanies your visualizations. This loss usually has to do with your fondness or familiarity, with the old behavior and with your realizing the need to let it go to effect the desired change. This sense of loss is a natural phenomenon, and we go through it whenever a change happens in our lives.

It is especially important that you acknowledge and feel your way through it. You may experience confusion about how you will handle yourself in a certain situation, being smoke-free. Simply see yourself in that situation being smoke free.

As Gary Craig of the Emotional Freedom Techniques calls them "The Horrible How's" leave them alone and simply see yourself in that situation being smoke free.

When these situations come up, particularly when you visualize, you can choose to rely on your creative ability to find a satisfactory outcome to the situation. It is important to always know that if you choose to act and react the old way, no one forced you into that behavior.

Since you used your creative ability to develop one behavior, do the same process and simply change the result. The saying, *it is as easy or hard as you choose to make it*, is an absolute truth. You can choose the thoughts you have about the level of easiness involved in any situation that you are involved in.

It is important that you believe the truth that you have absolute control over your thoughts, actions, and reactions. This concept must be imbedded in your head. You really must believe this idea before it can work. It allows you to become responsible for who you are.

By owning responsibility for your actions, and accepting the fact that you have ultimate control over who you are and how you act/behave, that puts you in a position to effect change. This change is another message. The old message of how hard it is going to be for you not to smoke can be replaced with this brand-new message:

Not smoking is the easiest thing I have ever done

By choosing to repeat this message regularly throughout the day, you can make a new and lasting impression on your belief system that will replace the old one. Remember that at one time in your life you had ***no*** thought about cigarettes, only to develop factual and opinionated false information about smoking and/or being smoke free.

You have chosen a date to stop smoking because you love yourself. See yourself as a non-smoker and you use your creative ability to get yourself through old behavioral pictures of you smoking. Now, you reinforce them all with the statement *Not smoking is the easiest thing I have ever done or being smoke free is easy for me.* Notice that all the action being taken is in your head—all the conflict is in your head because you are still smoking.

Every day you are constantly working on yourself to see, hear, and sense new information about yourself. This new statement could be used many times throughout the day. The more it is used, the faster it will impress your mind and the sooner you will demonstrate the new behavior. Please realize that whenever we deny something, we are affirming something else. So, to show an external change, we begin the process by effecting the change internally.

All these new messages you choose to give yourself allow you to be a non-smoker internally first, which is where it must happen. You can sense within yourself how you act, react, feel, smell, taste, dress, and behave as a non-smoker. By going through the work internally first, by designing your new life as you want it to be first, this enables you to flow naturally most easily into a new behavior. When you accept that it is the inside change that makes for the external manifestation, our work becomes easier.

THERE IS a direct flow from thought to action. This flow is demonstrated every day of your life. Become aware of this law at work, see it, sense it, and flow with it. You have the control. *Not smoking is the easiest thing I have ever done.* Repeat it until you know you believe it.

It is necessary that you love yourself enough to take charge of your life. Self-love means that you care enough about yourself to demonstrate the new behavior or behaviors. It is being consistent in thought and action. This negates the conflict and allows for a flow. Since you do not smoke for others, you will not quit for others. You are choosing to quit for yourself, since you are the only one who ultimately matters when it comes to these changes in behavior, anyway. Self-love also symbolizes the willingness to take charge of your life, which enables you to drop excuses for not changing things about yourself.

You want to change, in other words, no procrastination. If you love yourself, really love yourself, then acting on the exercises and the ultimate demonstration of not smoking will easily happen. For several weeks now you have shown the willingness to take charge of your thought-life. You have given yourself messages you may not have believed, but you allowed yourself to repeat them regularly. These actions all show that you can change at will if only you put energy into it.

Look now at the changes that have happened to you the last few weeks you have been involved in this course. How do you feel today about the new messages? Are they as foreign to you? Do you feel more comfortable with them? Do you notice a difference inside you? Is it easier for you to tell yourself these new things about yourself than when you first started?

These changes show the transformations on the subconscious level, and the alterations have taken place. Like I said at the beginning, the subconscious does not know the difference between fact or fiction. It just accepts what you tell it and produces the results.

Everyone has an automatic success mechanism built in (*Psycho-Cybernetics*). This helps you keep on course and get what you have focused your attention on. Your singleness of purpose, of choosing to be smoke free, adds fuel to the emotional fire necessary to propel you to the successful completion of your goal. Your mind creates the entire scene, just as you want it to be. Know now that you are the one in absolute control of your being smoke free. It is always up to you. What is happening is you have begun to consciously take control of your life. You are in control. God gave us free will to use in whatever way we saw fit. What is going on is you are exercising your will in a different way.

Instead of using your will power to tell you in thought, picture, and action that you can't not smoke because of your many excuses, you now have used your will power to tell you in thought, picture, and action that you choose to be smoke free (easily and effortlessly). You are not using any different energy, only redirecting the energy you now expend and are having it go in a different direction—it is a choice, remember?

AS YOU REPEAT the new messages daily, then the behavior simply changes with no effort on your part. Follow the instructions and see what comes up for you.

CHAPTER 5

So far, we have gone over the following:

- Deciding for a positive reason
- Setting a goal, you believe you can achieve
- Seeing yourself as a non-smoker and enjoying yourself in this new image
- Telling yourself that, "You now choose to be smoke free. *Being smoke free is the easiest thing you have ever done."*

All these new messages are now being backed with action. Since you started reading this book you have been taking the action by reinforcing the new behavior daily through thought. From this point on, you will now follow through by stopping smoking on the date you said you would stop smoking. By putting enough energy into this mental step, now the physical action of not smoking is a simple formality. You started the course with this purpose, didn't you, that you wanted to stop smoking?

How you believe about yourself, and what action you take on that this belief is the driving force behind you. Let's be truly clear on this principle. Get in touch now with the strength of the belief of you as a smoker, then that of you being a non-smoker. Which carries the most weight? Why do you think that is so? Because it is the message that you tell yourself the most often. This is the message you take the action on most frequently. To know which way it came out for you is particularly important.

If the message is more prone to be still in smoking, then you know you simply must take more time with the exercises. If it is stronger to see you as a non-smoker, then be assured that your psyche is believing the messages about you as-a non-smoker that you have been feeding it. This self-awareness continues to play an important part in this entire change process.

Now, it is incredibly significant that you get in touch with how powerful you are as a person. It is important to realize now, as never before, that you are the one who shapes your destiny. As you believe this more and more, and the only way you will believe it, is by telling yourself this as well as by seeing yourself in the solution.

This idea, as you practice it, will transform your entire life. The singleness of purpose you have regarding stopping smoking gives you the type of tunnel vision necessary for you to propel yourself to the successful completion of your goal. You are seeing yourself successfully completing this tangible goal, and by feeding the solution daily as often as possible, by countering all defeating messages with solution messages, you will surely succeed. Because you get what you think about the most.

Since you have a choice in what you affirm about yourself, then continue to affirm that *Being smoke free is the easiest thing*

I have ever done. Affirm regularly that you are relaxed and at ease without a cigarette. That you are at your desired weight, that you have a pleasant personality, that you have plenty to do with your hands, that you really enjoy being with yourself as a non-smoker.

Affirmations are with you throughout the day, anyway, so consciously choose more positive ones. Simply be the kind of person you want to be. You are in control of your habit, which is a part of your life. I say and believe *The most difficult part of all of this is to see that the work is all in your head* (*mind*). *All these teachings deal with this intangible world. We are dealing with an intangible reality, that of your mind.* (Do you understand this?)

The mind manifests its thoughts in the physical world and operates under the same laws as the tangible world, but people do not seem to treat it the same. We cannot easily see the changes in thoughts as they are developing. We can tire of, or lose interest, because we do not have physical results to hold on to as quickly as when doing tangible projects. So, you need to understand that the changes do, in fact, occur if you will work at and be patient until the desired result is demonstrated in the new behavior. The reason I go to yesterday's behavior and compare it with the new behavior is to help you see that you have used this process already. Today you choose your reality. You are not a victim, you are the creator of your life.

So, if you are the master of your life, then effect the desired change at will as you have effected a change in every other area of your life. Notice the time element for yourself to change any behavior of yours. Isn't it true that for some things, the change happens immediately, and for other internal changes, it seems we wrestle with them forever? For the easy ones, we are simply not that attached to the behavior, so it is no big deal to let it go. But, for the harder ones, we must let go of a complete belief system: how we live our life, who we are with, how our house is decorated, what we think about—all the messages, endless, how we want to change ... But...

This *But* is the catch. If we continue to use *But,* we are holding on to the old and refusing to accept the new. Be aware, you have learned how to counter the *But,* and as you use the counter messages and see the desired solution, then you can get rid of the *But's.* This conflict makes books like this and others necessary. We all get caught up in many ineffective belief systems and build a rationale around why we are the victim of the situation and how we would like to change but cannot because... and so on.

I learned about this term recently, and it seems to apply. The term *Confirmational bias* states, "We get a narrative in our mind about what we feel/think/imagine is happening, self-talk about being smoke free for instance, the narrative could arise from a preexisting belief, a theory developed based on other things we have seen, or from what someone tells us we are seeing/experiencing. Then, we look for information that confirms that what we are seeing, experiencing corresponds with that narrative, and We don't play devil's advocate with ourselves by searching for things that would contradict that narrative." Taken in part from the movie "What the Bleep" and then my expansion on the idea.

So, a book like this enables us to stop long enough and examine our beliefs and behavior, and through this process we can choose to see how we can act on the choice and develop the new desired behavior.

- The book has helped you to facilitate your stopping a thought and action and change directions
- You decided you did not want to smoke

- You are willing to stop the old mental and visual messages with new mental and visual messages

It is you who will finally choose to believe the new message about yourself regarding smoking: *Stopping is the easiest thing I have ever done.* It is easy to do, but it is initially hard to believe you can do it.

A lot of things in life are like this. The processes we talked about are as follows:

- Goal setting
- Decision making for a positive reason
- Visualization
- Creative imagination
- Action

These things are already in use in every area of your life. Remember, once you have identified an area in your life you want to change, decide what date you want to change it by, feel how intense you are about expecting the change, imagine you as the new type of person you want to become, then reinforce these messages daily.

Put it into action. It is your life. You know you do have control and you are already exercising control in the present behavior.

THESE EXERCISES GIVE you another way of looking at an old belief system and putting a different belief system into play without having to fight at all. The key seems to be in not fighting. There is no requirement to believe the new information at first, just to see it and to say it. Simply allow the new belief time to be accepted. Therefore, the messages need to be seen and heard multiple times every day, why it is important to see yourself as a non-smoker enjoying yourself, to especially not judge you for smoking or not smoking or anyone else.

As the new, or different, messages are repeated daily, then the behavior simply changes with no effort on your part. All you need to do are the exercises. Bring the mind, and the body will follow. Follow the instructions and take what you get.

In a nutshell, what I am saying is, take control of your thought-life. Your thoughts show themselves in actions. So, by constantly noticing your thoughts and changing the ones that do not positively benefit you, you will then show behavior in your life that will help you achieve any goal or idea you set your mind on.

CHAPTER 6

Guarantee

I guarantee you will never smoke again. This guarantee, like all other guarantees, has conditions that must be met:

- You tell yourself and act on the choice—*you choose to be smoke* free.
- See yourself as non-smoker daily enjoying yourself.
- Whenever, if ever you want a cigarette, do anything but light up.

Being Smoke Free is easy for me

Write down what attaches you to smoking

1. Write down why your life will be worse off when you stop.

These are the preoccupations you are attached to that enable you to smoke and have problems related to being smoke free.

For example: *I will be nervous, anxious, and get fat. I will not be able to sleep. I'll get bored. I'll have no one to talk with. I won't know how to be or what to after meals. I will not know how to in the car or on the phone. After sex will be awkward, etc.*

2. Write down why you think your life will be better.

For example: *My health will improve. I will breathe better. I will save money. I can be around non-smoking friends and family members. I will be more socially accepted.*

3. Write down your triggers for lighting up, or chewing tobacco? "

For example: *Waking up, in the car, with coffee, with alcohol, to break tension, stress relief, after sex, handle emotions, when I anxious, nervous, annoyed, etc.*

BONUS CHAPTER

In 1990, I learned about this simple process that helps anyone who does it to effect any change more easily and effortlessly in their life.

- It is simple to do, and you will only get a benefit from it, or not. It can only help, never hurts anyone.
- It comes from the wisdom found in Chinese medicine and is around 6,000 years old.
- It works with the meridians, or energy pathways, in the body.

Meridians carry life force energy, arteries carry life-giving blood. When one withholds emotions like fear, anxiety, anger, resentment, shame, excitement, joy, sadness, etc. The energy of the thought builds up and the body feels this block. Like a nervous stomach when our self-esteem is threatened or problems with mobility when our core beliefs are rigid, etc.

Roger Callahan (www.tfttapping.com), and Gary Craig of *Emotional Freedom Techniques* (www.emofree.com), are two people to study if you are interested in learning more about this amazing process.

These are just the basics here with little to no information about the meridians because I want to use the tool to help you overcome any anxiety or self-doubt you may have. The above-mentioned references can give you volumes to read about. The tapping points are numbered and are to be done in the sequence laid out for you.

First, rate your level of doubt, disbelief, discomfort, fear about doing this Smoking Cessation Thing on a scale from 0 no doubt, disbelief, discomfort, fear discomfort, to 10 massive amounts of doubt, disbelief, discomfort, fear , etc.

Next, notice in your body where you feel this discomfort. Is it soft, hard, mushy, hot, cold, round, oblong, big, little, etc.? Now the light tapping sequences.

1. Karate chop (fatty part of the side of the one hand chopping down on the palm of the other hand). Tap five times saying, "Even though I am going to be smoke-free, and I am unsure about it does not mean that I have to be nervous or unsure about it." You could also say: "Just because I am unsure of myself and my ability to maintain my being Smoke Free does not mean I will have problems being smoke free." Say anything else to define and dispute the problem.
2. Move to the upper left chest to a tender spot an inch below the Adams apple and two inches out from the sternum, that is tender. Tap five times saying, "I deeply and profoundly accept myself whether I am a smoker or not." You could also say, "I deeply and profoundly accept myself smoking or not."

3. Now, move to the center of the top of your head. Tap five times saying, "In order for any new ideas, beliefs, behaviors to come in, I must create a space for them to be." You could also say, "I now create a blank space within me to receive the new ideas and behaviors."
4. Now move to along the eyebrows. Tap five times saying, "I open up see, hear, listen to my intuition to give me the answers I need to accomplish the task of my getting and remaining smoke free."
5. Next, move to the side of the eyes and state "I forgive ________________. They did their best, and although it was not very good, it was their best. I release them with forgiveness and love for my benefit not theirs." You could also say, "I forgive myself for my nicotine habit. It was the best I could do, but it was not very good, and I release me for my benefit."
6. Next, tap under the eyes on the bone, tap five times saying, "My anxiety is of my own creation because I try to live in the future, a time that does not now or ever will exist. NOW is the totality of all time, and it is the only time that exists. For me to be in present time all I need to do is look down at me feet and see them standing there and I am in the present moment."
7. Now, tap under the nose and say, "Shame is a lie has always been a lie and will always be a lie. The only life it has is the life I give it and I now withdraw all meanings I have associated with it in the past."
8. Now, tap under the nose. This is the spot for toxic shame saying, "regardless of how much shame/pain

I have endured, by how I internalized my story about my life events, how big the mountain of shame is, does not mean that it is true. It just means that is how I have internalized it with no factual information attached to it." You can also say, "I built this mountain of shame I alone can destroy or dispute it and I am willing to destroy it."

9. Next, tap five times on the kidney meridians which are located on the upper chest, one inch below the Adams apple and two inches to either side of the sternum. Saying, "I now create within me an internal protective container that houses the guilt, shame, muck and mess of all my dysfunctional beliefs and behaviors. It gathers in the container and when full, it goes down my body, stomach, knees, calves, feet and out of my body deep into the earth so no one will be able to step in it." Repeat the above two more times.
10. Now, tap five times on your sides four inches down from your armpit saying, "I now stand for myself regardless of the difficulties I may have, regardless of level of disbelief in this process or my ability to successfully stop and maintain m smoke free behavior."
11. Repeat the above 10 steps one more time then rate your level of discomfort on your 1-10 scale with your thought of being able to stop and stay stopped smoking.
12. Repeat until the level of difficulty is at a 0. Tap 8 to 12 times a day, or a total of six minutes a day until you notice there is no discomfort with the smoking cessation thought. When you mentally or physically put yourself in a smoking situation, or

> when you are experiencing a smoking trigger and feel you are a smoker, simply affirm you are a non-smoker and it is easy and effortless for you.

This simple process can and does help you release any anxiety, fear, resistance you may have to stopping and remain smoke free.

Like I said, this a BONUS. The main process discussed in the previous chapters are the reports of action taken to successfully product the result of being smoke free, easy for me and countless others from 1979 till now.

BIBLIOGRAPHY

Rolling Thunder by Doug Boyd

As A Man Thinketh by James Allen

The Silva Method by Jose Silva

Psycho-Cybernetics by Maxwell Maltz and Dan Kennedy

Creative Visualization by Shakti Gawain

Thought Field Therapy by Roger Callahan

Emotional Freedom Techniques by Gary Craig

ABOUT THE AUTHOR

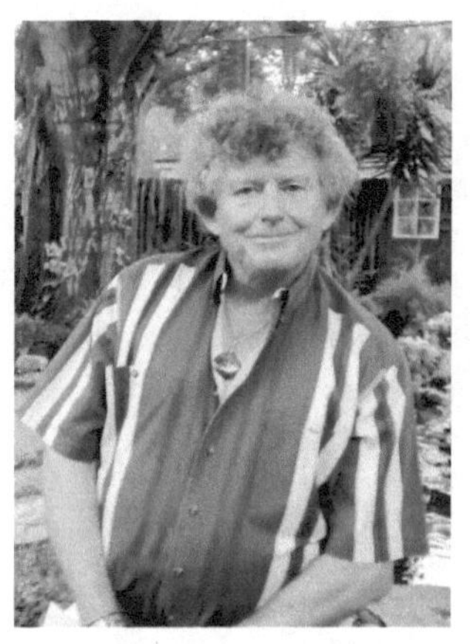

In 1973, I became a therapist in the addiction recovery field after I got off drugs, including alcohol. In 1979 I stopped a 4.5 pack a day cigarette habit. This smoking cessation program I developed has helped thousands of people stop and stay stopped since then.

Over my career, I have functioned as a therapist, Program Director, Clinical Staff Trainer, Continuing Education Hour Educator and in 1989 started a holistic private practice.

I've learned many Western therapy skills, Cognitive Behavioral Therapy, Hypnosis, Therapeutic Massage, Voice Dialogue, Motivational Enhancement, The Silva Method, etc., and Chinese medicine and rapid healing techniques like Auricular Acupuncture, Acupressure EFT, and TFT, Brain Spotting, EMDR, ART, Polyvegal Therapy, etc.

 facebook.com/michael.yeager.39948

 linkedin.com/in/michael-yeager-8b95762

www.ingramcontent.com/pod-product-compliance
Lightning Source LLC
LaVergne TN
LVHW050944080826
845145LV00004B/1410

* 9 7 8 1 9 4 0 3 8 5 3 9 6 *